Rheumatoid Arthritis Pain Relief

Wendy Owen

HH Dip (H.H.T

Disclaimer

CONTENTS

INTRODUCTION

If you have rheumatoid arthritis and are looking to decrease your pain medication, or are hoping for a remission, then I may be able to help. If you are trying to have more control over the disease and your health in general, then I can help you. If you simply want to prevent rheumatoid arthritis or other immune disorders then this could be the book for you. I have tried to keep the language in this book as simple and easy to understand as possible, so it's easy to read.

I have no formal medical training. My area of expertise is in natural and holistic medicine. I have a Diploma in Holistic Health Therapy. Holistic health basically means looking at the body as a whole and healing disease at the source. I have put a full disclaimer at the end of the book. Please feel free to contact me if you would like a copy of the disclaimer in advance or if you would like to verify my diploma :

wendy@rheumatoidarthritisfacts.org

Although no-one seems to be able to agree on the exact causes of rheumatoid arthritis, it's now generally accepted in medical circles that it's an auto-immune disease. What triggers the immune system to react in this way is still undecided, but what is clear is treating the immune system can help rheumatoid arthritis and even create a state of remission.

Is there a cure?

The medical profession says there is no cure. However if you can achieve permanent remission, it's as good as a cure in my opinion. I used to have this disease but I haven't had any symptoms for a couple of years. It may come back, but I doubt it, because I keep my immune system in peak condition which keeps any symptoms at bay.

I had aches and pains that couldn't be explained away for any physical reason. All the X rays and scans showed no abnormalities. I had a blood test for the rheumatoid arthritis gene, which came back negative. My doctor didn't exactly say it was all in my head, but I got that impression. I sought a second opinion and was diagnosed with rheumatoid arthritis in the summer of 2009.

It was not a particularly severe form of the disease, however the symptoms were bad enough to have to take medication. This was enough to motivate me to explore more natural ways to alleviate pain, but most of all, to come up with a way to get rid of the symptoms for good. My training in holistic health gave me a good start and six months later I had no pain or inflammation in my body at all.

Everything I did is laid out here. Some of the things suggested in this book I didn't use, because I didn't have to. However they are well documented as good natural treatments for rheumatoid arthritis and I have included them.

This is not a book on herbal remedies, although I have included a few of the better ones for the sake of completeness. This is a book on how to get your immune system into a healthy state where it can perform the task it needs to do, which is to ward off viruses, while leaving healthy body tissue intact.

Read on to get rid of arthritis pain…

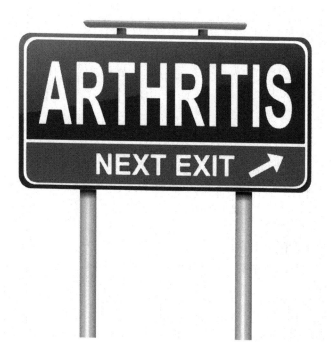

WHAT IS AN AUTO-IMMUNE DISEASE?

Rheumatoid arthritis is almost certainly an auto-immune disease. There's a lot of speculation about what causes rheumatoid arthritis, but more and more, research is pointing to the fact that it's an immune system malfunction that causes rheumatoid arthritis.

So what's an auto-immune disease? It's a condition that cause the immune system to attack and destroy its own tissues. There are several kinds of immune disease; Rheumatoid Arthritis, Lupus, Chron's Disease, Multiple Sclerosis and Guillain-Barre Syndrome among others.

To put it simply, auto-immune diseases can be described as a break-down of communication between our body's cells. Our immune cells can no longer distinguish between harmful invaders and our own body tissue. In the past these diseases were believed to be mainly caused by peoples' genes, however more and more evidence is emerging that says lifestyle and environmental factors are more likely to be the culprits.

Women succumb to auto-immune diseases more frequently than men for reasons that are still vague. Several theories have been put forward - there may be a biological link or it could simply be a lifestyle issue as women tend to be under more stress through multitasking by having full time jobs and raising a family at the same time. It could also be hormonal.

Where is the immune system?

Your immune system is composed of your digestive tract, body tissues, blood and the linings of your nose and mouth. Special "scout" cells can isolate foreign molecules attempting to enter your body and head them off. Once these scout cells find a foreign invader like a virus, they call in other immune cells to destroy the offending virus. This is how a healthy immune system protects us from disease.

When the immune system is compromised, however, it isn't able to discern between the foreign invaders and your own tissues. In the case of rheumatoid arthritis, the immune system targets the joint linings, or synovium for reasons that are not yet understood. This leads to redness, pain, inflammation and in severe cases, the joints themselves can become deformed. This is why an early diagnosis is so crucial.

So why does our friendly immune system suddenly become the enemy? Well there are several reasons, many of which are under our control and we'll talk about these in the next chapter.

Points to take away:

-Rheumatoid arthritis is an auto-immune disease.

-It is caused by the immune system attacking joints and surrounding tissues.

-Auto-immune diseases can be controlled by healing the immune system.

WHAT CAUSES THE IMMUNE SYSTEM TO REBEL?

Auto-immune diseases can be triggered by many things. Some are lifestyle issues that we can control, others are environmental factors that we have no direct control over, but we can minimize the effects.

When the immune system is alerted to an injury or attack from viruses or bacteria, it triggers inflammation in that area. Inflammation is a normal defense mechanism of the body and protects us from bacteria entering through a wound, or from diseases such as the flu and other even more deadly illnesses. This type of inflammation is called "acute" and is necessary for us to survive.

Chronic inflammation is when the normal immune response doesn't switch off. When inflammation is chronic, it can trigger an alarming array of diseases which include rheumatoid arthritis. This is the reason those who suffer with this disease have red swollen and painful joints. The immune system is attacking its own tissues.

Chronic Inflammation is probably one of our worst health enemies today! So what causes it?

Toxic overload

These days we are bombarded from every angle with toxins, chemicals and mold. We are exposed in our homes, our workplaces and even outside in the garden. The body was never equipped to deal with the level of chemicals that attack it daily, so it attempts to store the chemicals it's unable to dispose of in our fat cells. These chemicals can literally stay there for decades and are one of the main reasons why so many people find it hard to lose weight. The body needs your adipose (fat) tissues as a storage bin and is not likely to let go of them without a fight!

There are many things we can do to prevent toxic overload and minimize our exposure to it and we'll look further into this in another chapter.

Stress

Most people realize stress is a leading cause of disease in our modern world - some researchers say it can cause up to 80% of diseases. While a small amount of stress is fine, too much becomes debilitating and can cause lack of sleep, emotional distress and (you've guessed it!) an overloaded immune system.

Poor diet

One of our best defenses against all kinds of diseases is the food we eat and (perhaps more importantly) don't eat. We can use food as medicine for our bodies if we know about nutrition and prevent a whole host of diseases, including cancer and of course, auto immune diseases such as rheumatoid arthritis and diabetes.

Not eating enough healthy foods and especially eating too many unhealthy foods is a leading cause of inflammation and immune disorders. We'll explore what to eat and not to eat and what supplements are good for rheumatoid arthritis further on in this book.

Food intolerance

This surprises many people, but eating a food that you have intolerance towards can lead to an immune reaction every time you eat it. This of course leads to inflammation and the usual downward spiral. The thing is, some people may be intolerant to a food that's considered healthy. To make things more complicated they may be totally unaware that they have this intolerance. Aarrrgh!

The most common foods that cause these types of reactions are wheat (gluten intolerance) and milk (lactose or casein intolerance). As always, we'll expand more about this in another chapter.

Genetics

This was thought to be the main reason people developed auto-immune disorders. Although it's still considered in some medical quarters as the main reason, there is overwhelming evidence that it's our lifestyle and environment that play a far larger part in this equation than our genes do. This is a good thing as it gives us some control over our health!

How do I know if I have chronic inflammation?

It's quite easy. Just ask your doctor for a blood test that can measure *C-reactive protein.* This will measure the degree of chronic inflammation in your body. This is an important test and one you should not put off.

Points to take away:

-Chronic inflammation is a cause of immune diseases.

-Stress can lead to chronic inflammation.

-Toxic overload weakens the immune system.

-A poor diet and food intolerance can also cause chronic inflammation.

-Genes are not as important as once thought as a cause of auto-immune diseases.

-A blood test can measure chronic inflammation.

TOXIC OVERLOAD!

There are many things that can upset an otherwise healthy immune system, and one of the worst is toxic overload. When immune systems were invented all those years ago, they simply weren't designed to cope with the chemical load our bodies have to cope with in this modern day and age ☺

So what are these toxins? How do they get into our body and how do they upset the immune system?

Toxins are chemicals, bacteria and viruses and they can enter our body through the mouth, nose, eyes and skin.

Those that enter through the mouth are mainly contained in food and medications. Our immune systems are well equipped to handle bacteria and viruses; however chemicals and processed foods are a different story. When these enter the digestive tract, they are accosted by the cells in the intestinal lining. Over time these cells become weakened and the intestinal lining becomes inflamed.

The following is a list of potential irritants:

Refined and processed foods

These can affect us in two ways. First, if we eat too many refined (highly processed) and not enough raw and whole foods it can affect the balance of bacteria in the gut. This leads to an over-abundance of unhealthy bacteria. Second, refined carbohydrates can contain toxic molds.

Antibiotics

Antibiotics can also cause an imbalance in the ratio of healthy to unhealthy bacteria.

Caffeine and Alcohol

These are fine in small doses but continual use over long periods of time can irritate the gut lining.

Flavorings and colorants

These are found mainly in processed food. Preservatives can also upset the delicate intestinal lining.

We were just not designed to eat these things and although some people seem to be able to get away with it, others can't and may develop a complaint called "leaky gut syndrome". It doesn't sound very pleasant and it isn't!

Leaky gut is where a damaged intestinal wall allows molecules of undigested food, yeasts and other toxins to leak into the bloodstream. This in turn causes the liver to try and eliminate these wastes from the blood.

Unfortunately the liver was never intended to do so much extra work which means many of these toxins remain in the body. This causes an immune response followed by inflammation. If this goes on unchecked day after day, chronic inflammation is the result, leaving us prone to auto immune disorders, including (you've guessed it) rheumatoid arthritis.

Fortunately there are things we can do to repair a leaky gut and we'll cover that in the chapter on enzymes.

Food allergies

This is a largely ignored cause of immune system disorders. If you are allergic to a certain food, each time you eat that food, yes even a healthy food, it will trigger an immune response and therefore inflammation.

How do you know what foods you may be allergic to? You will probably experience uncomfortable symptoms such as cramping or bloating, however you may not know what food is causing it. Food allergies are very common and some people may have a food allergy without realizing it.

Points to take away:

-Toxins from our food or from the environment can cause immune reactions and lead to auto-immune disease.

-Eating a food to which we are intolerant, can cause chronic inflammation of the intestinal lining and leaky gut syndrome.

-Eating a poor diet composed largely of processed foods can also lead to chronic inflammation.

WHAT ELSE TRIGGERS OUR IMMUNE SYSTEMS?

Chemicals in the home

Your home can be a virtual chemical storage facility. Consider how many cleaning products you use. Most of these are chemical based and some of them are quite potent! While most of us are careful not to touch cleaning products with our bare hands, they can pollute the air in our home and we can inhale them without realizing it.

Some of the worst of these are drain cleaners, toilet cleaners and oven cleaners, but even the humble all-purpose spray cleaners can affect our immune system. Do yourself a favor and make your own green cleaning products or you can buy chemical free cleaners and detergents on line, or in health stores.

Insecticides are another health hazard. Although they are designed to kill insects and not humans, anything with the power to kill has some pretty nasty stuff in it! If you must use them, try not to inhale and leave the room as soon as you can.

New carpets, paint and new car interiors are other sources of chemicals that spread through the air in our homes and cars. Air fresheners that we spray around the home may smell like nature, however they're usually anything but!

Chemicals in the atmosphere

This is largely out of our control, especially if we live and work in the city. These toxins come mostly from motor vehicles and factory emissions. These can also enter the water supply, so we not only get to inhale them, but to drink them as well.

Beauty products

If you've ever read the label on some of these products it probably turned your brain to mush and you decided it was all too much to worry about. Here's the thing - you don't need all those fancy ingredients in your beauty products. Most of them won't make you look younger and you will save a lot of money from simply making your own cosmetics or buying natural ones from the health food store.

Why are these "cosmeceuticals" so expensive? Because you are paying for the fancy container, the advertising and the brand name! The only thing I *do* spend a bit of money on is a good sunscreen from the health store. This doesn't contain chemicals but screens the sun using "invisible" zinc. There's no chemicals that can enter your pores and disrupt your immune system.

Can using store bought cosmetics really cause immune problems? Put it this way. Our bodies are already struggling to cope with this modern toxic overload, whatever you can do to lessen the load will help.

Start by doing this bit by bit. You can start by eliminating certain toxic foods from your diet. Next begin replacing your cleaners with natural products. Speaking of diet, we will be addressing that in the next chapter.

By now you're probably wishing you'd never started reading this chapter! But take heart, nearly every toxic solution has an answer. You just have to take it gradually. How do you eat an elephant? One bite at a time!

Points to take away:

-Chemicals can be found in the home as well as in the atmosphere.

-Your skin care products and cosmetics may be causing immune issues.

-We can't control chemicals in the atmosphere, but we can strengthen our immune system to cope.

DIET - LET'S END THE CONFUSION!

There are probably two main things to remember about a diet for rheumatoid arthritis. One is what to eat and the other is what NOT to eat. The latter may actually be more important!

When dealing with auto-immune disorders, what you put into your body is critical. It's vital to feed the immune system the right nutrients it needs for repair. These days it's difficult to do this with food alone unless you consume a raw food diet. This is challenging for most of us who are in our comfort zone where food is concerned! However it is possible to do and something to try if you are interested.

The food we eat today (raw or cooked), is not as wholesome as it was thirty to forty years ago. This is due to depleted soils, pesticide use and long storage times. There are ways around this; you can grow your own vegetables or you can buy organic produce. The latter is a lot easier, if you are financially able to do so, as it is more expensive to buy organically grown produce.

The best thing to do when changing your eating habits is to take a break from food for a few days. Many natural doctors recommend this for rheumatoid arthritis sufferers. It can help reduce swelling, inflammation and pain quite significantly. This may be due to the body starting to detoxify itself, taking stress off the organs such as the liver and pancreas.

Fasting gives the digestive system a bit of rest and relaxation after working up to 18 hours a day! Many people go on fasts before embarking on a weight loss program. Others go on a fast one day per week. It's best to check with your health practitioner though, as some people have medical conditions that make fasting unsuitable.

The classic fast is to drink water only and not to eat any food whatsoever. It's important, if you decide to do this, to take it easy and not exert yourself too much. Your body will be low on energy, but you may start to feel much better after a day or two. It's possible that you may indeed feel worse for a little while due to the detoxification process.

A less drastic way to detoxify is to go on a juice fast. Juice fasting can be done for slightly longer, as you are taking in some nutrients. There are many good books on juicing and many recipes on the internet too. Most healthy juices are a combination of vegetables and fruit. It's best not to add too much fruit as you will be taking in excess fructose.

You can drink some juice every hour if you need to or you can have three or four an hour - whatever you find suits you best. Make sure you have all your ingredients on hand before beginning a fast, as you won't want to have to go shopping in the middle of a fast and be tempted by the sight of yummy food!

So what **should** you eat on an arthritis diet?

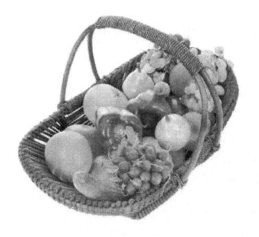

Generally speaking a healthy diet which includes a good variety of fresh foods is best. There are some people who have an adverse reaction to nightshade foods, which include eggplants, tomatoes, potatoes and peppers as these contain alkaloids which can make rheumatoid arthritis symptoms worse. However only certain individuals react to these foods and it's not a good idea to give them up altogether unless you're sure they **do** affect you.

Cooking nightshade foods can lower the alkaloid content. I would advise doing this with tomatoes as they have an important antioxidant called lycopene which is best released when cooked.

People with rheumatoid arthritis often have trouble eating meat and other animal produce. Red meat tends to make rheumatoid arthritis symptoms worse in certain individuals. Again before giving up red meat for good, try cutting it out for a couple of months to see if your symptoms improve. If they do, then substitute fish and chicken and vegetable proteins such as lentils for your protein requirements.

Dairy foods are another potential problem. It's extremely common for adults to have intolerance to lactose; however the milk protein casein is another cause of intolerance. As with meat, you can try cutting dairy out for a couple of weeks also and see the result. There are some good milk substitutes on the market, such as oat milk and almond milk. Soy milk is the most common alternative; however some people are sensitive to soy products.

Some people may have milk intolerance but find they can eat cheese without a problem. It's just a matter of testing. You can also buy soy cheese and it tastes a lot better than it sounds ☺

Acid and alkaline foods

Some nutritionists believe that certain foods are more acidic than others. Examples of extreme acid foods are meat and dairy products. Alkaline food include vegetables, fruits and nuts. Acidic foods can put a huge strain on our body and cause leaching of valuable minerals from our bones, such as calcium and magnesium, in order to try and alkalize the blood.

This predisposes us to fatigue and a range of health problems, including chronic disease. This is a very simplified explanation I have given here, so do further research if you would like to find further information on acid and alkaline foods. Don't cut out whole food groups without knowing exactly what you are doing first. If in doubt, consult a nutritionist.

Celiac disease and wheat

Celiac disease is more than a food intolerance or allergy; it is a dangerous condition that can make people very sick. There has been a connection made between celiac disease and auto-immune diseases such as rheumatoid arthritis.

People with celiac disease experience unpleasant digestive symptoms when eating foods made with wheat. This includes a huge range of foods as we are not just talking about bread, pasta and breakfast cereals. Many foods contain wheat flour such as gravy mix, MSG (monosodium glutamate), which is sometimes used as a flavoring for Asian dishes, soy sauce, some store bought hamburgers, baked beans and even some of the cheaper chocolate brands.

The ingredient called gluten that is found mainly in wheat, but also in rye and barley is the problem. Oats in themselves do not contain gluten, but are sometimes contaminated with wheat flour in the manufacturing process. As you can see it's a minefield out there!

The good news is that there are many gluten-free foods on the market today. No longer do celiac sufferers have to bake their own bread! However it is tricky to identify all the foods that contain hidden gluten and you may have to read the label on any product you buy. The internet is a good source of information on where to get gluten-free foods, such as rice, pasta and bread made from gluten-free grains.

If you suspect that gluten may be a problem for you, go to the doctor and have some tests done. Don't stop eating gluten foods before you do this as the tests will be inconclusive.

There are other real diet taboos too - these are for everyone, not just those suffering with rheumatoid arthritis. Some of them may surprise you. This is because they tend to go against mainstream nutritional advice.

Canola oil

Ever heard of a Canola plant? No? That's because it doesn't exist. Canola oil is made from the seed of the Rape plant. The Rape plant is toxic for insects and we humans simply can't digest it. The British used Canola oil to feed their livestock around 20 years ago and had to stop due to the shocking health problems it caused.

Rapeseed oil is irradiated to form Canola oil and the food industry claims it is healthy because it is an unsaturated fat. It is not healthy. Most of the other vegetable oils don't do too much for you either. They are all omega 6 fats and although we do need some omega 6 in our diet, we usually get far too much especially if we eat pre-cooked foods such as fish and chips or baked goods. Stick to olive oil for your salads, coconut oil for cooking and butter for your toast. If you're worried about your weight, just go easy on these. Leave polyunsaturated oils where they belong, which is anywhere but on your plate.

Margarine

They are still advertising this tasteless goo in Australia. Margarine contains trans-fats and it's artificially produced. All trans-fats are toxic for the body. Fortunately most countries have to declare them on the label. Just have a small amount of butter instead - it tastes better anyway!

So what *are* the best foods for a rheumatoid arthritis diet?

Basically a diet comprising a variety of vegetables, fruits, chicken, fish and whole grains is the best way to eat when you have rheumatoid arthritis. There is no set menu, although having said that, there are certain foods that have special health benefits:

Spinach

This miracle green plant contains vitamins, essential fatty acids and anti-oxidants and also *salicylic acid*, which is natural pain reliever. Salicylic acid is the main ingredient of aspirin, but you won't get the side effects of aspirin from eating spinach. What spinach can do is get rid of inflammation in a safe and natural way.

Spinach also contains beta carotene (a precursor of vitamin A), vitamins E and C and vitamin K. Vitamin K is known to strengthen bone and cartilage while reducing inflammation in joints.

Spinach can be served in a salad or lightly cooked. Don't store it for too long or it will lose a lot of its nutritional value. If you can't buy fresh spinach, use the canned or frozen variety.

Pineapple

Pineapple contains an enzyme called *Bromelain* that can help ease joint and muscle pain. It is also a good source of vitamin C and manganese.

Kale

Kale is a healthy food source of calcium which, along with other minerals is important for bone strength, especially if you take rheumatoid arthritis medications. Why is this important? It's because taking calcium supplements is no longer advised by some medical specialists. Calcium in pill form can cause heart attacks according to recent research.

Calcium can also be found in almonds, tofu, sesame seeds and fish. Some canned fish have edible bones and this is where the highest concentration of calcium is found.

What about dairy? Dairy products can make rheumatoid arthritis symptoms worse in some people. Milk is also an acid causing food (along with red meat) which can leach calcium from bones.

Cherries

Cherries contain *anthocyanins* that fight inflammation and lower blood levels of uric acid, which can accumulate in the joints, causing pain. Below is an excerpt from NaturalNews.com (with permission):

A Michigan State University study found that "20 tart cherries were at least as effective as other painkilling remedies, including aspirin, ibuprofen, and other non-steroidal anti-inflammatory drugs (NSAIDs). That's why cherries are a popular folk remedy for arthritis and gout. Like many fruits and vegetables, cherries also have fiber and potassium - great snack".

Broccoli

Broccoli and its friends cauliflower, cabbage and Brussels sprouts contain a substance called *sulphorane*. Recent research claims that sulphorane can help block the effects of the Cox-2 enzyme which of one of the enzymes that cause joint inflammation. Typically NSAIDs are used to block Cox-2, but they do have serious side effects.

The greatest concentration of sulphorane is found in broccoli sprouts. But the adult vegetable still contains some. Cook lightly.

Green tea

Green tea is made from the same plant as black tea, except it is not fermented. This means it contains the most *polyphenols*. The polyphenol ECGC found in green tea is a powerful anti-oxidant which has healing properties that can protect against cancer, heart disease and rheumatoid arthritis. Four cups of green tea a day will possibly provide protection against cartilage damage and block the formation of prostaglandins which cause pain and inflammation.

Although green tea is still being tested on humans, there are no known side effects from drinking a few cups of green tea a day. So there is everything to gain and nothing to lose. Drink green tea on its own without milk and sugar.

Probiotics (good bacteria!)

It has been suggested that one of the causes of rheumatoid arthritis may be an imbalance of the micro flora in the intestines. Luckily we can correct this by consuming probiotics, either in food or by means of supplements.

<u>Probiotics are microscopic live bacteria that offset the bad bacteria we are exposed to from consuming alcohol, too much sugar and stress. Taking probiotics will keep the micro flora of the intestines in balance.</u>

Recent test have also uncovered some evidence that taking probiotics can even partially alleviate the symptoms of celiac disease.

Food sources of probiotics are yogurt and probiotic dairy drinks. A couple of non-dairy sources are pickled foods and tempeh (soy). A good brand of probiotic will contain 10 billion CFU of both *bifidobacteria* and *lactobacillus* species.

Points to take away:

-A rheumatoid arthritis diet is not set in cement and can be different for everyone.

-Eat a rainbow! Brightly colored fruits and vegetables contain lots of antioxidants.

-If it comes in a box it's probably best left in the box!

WHICH SUPPLEMENTS ARE BEST FOR RA?

I have included the best (in my opinion) supplements for rheumatoid arthritis pain relief here. These are not cures, they do however give relief to a lot of the painful symptoms. They are mostly without significant side effects. Some of them should not be taken with certain drugs so always check with your health care provider if you are on any medications.

Boswellia

Boswellia is an herb that has long been used in Ayurvedic medicine. It is sourced from a tree found in India (Boswellia Serrata). It has powerful anti-inflammatory properties which act by blocking inflammatory hormone like substances called *Leukotrienes* in the body.

Boswellia can significantly reduce pain, swelling and morning stiffness in those suffering from rheumatoid arthritis without the negative health effects of traditional anti-inflammatory medications, such as liver and kidney damage and stomach problems. Some people have been able to reduce their dosage of NSAIDs by taking Boswellia. This is significant, as NASAIDs can accelerate the destruction of cartilage, which is not at all helpful for people suffering from any type of arthritis.

Bromelain

Another potent anti-inflammatory - this time from the

pineapple. Bromelain can help those people on corticosteroid medication potentially reduce their dosage. This is good news as corticosteroid medications come with a range of side effects, including thinning of the bones, weight gain and cataracts. They are usually prescribed initially for acute arthritis symptoms and then tapered off gradually as these symptoms improve.

If you are using enzyme therapy as mentioned later in this book, bromelain may be a part of the enzymes you are already taking. If not, take 500 milligrams 3 times a day between meals. Check with your doctor if you are on any blood thinning medications before taking bromelain.

Omega 3 (fish oil or Krill oil)

Fish oil and Krill oil are well known for their anti-inflammatory properties and this is why a diet high in fish and low in meat is recommended for those with rheumatoid arthritis. These oils, known as Omega 3 oils EPA and DPA help to reduce inflammatory cytokines.

Omega 3 oils can also lower stress and anxiety which are known to increase inflammation in the body. They also have an immune balancing effect which is particularly helpful for those with rheumatoid arthritis.

Can we get enough Omega 3 by simply increasing the amount of fish in our diets? Probably, but only if we're young and healthy. For maximum benefits for rheumatoid arthritis, however, you would have to eat a ton of fish and that brings into play the problem of mercury toxicity as well. It's far better to take a high quality Omega 3 supplement that has been tested to contain no mercury.

I take Krill oil. It is better tolerated by the body and contains far less mercury than the larger fish from which fish oil is sourced. I take 1000 mg a day, down from 2000 mg. Some natural doctors advise taking higher doses, but check with your health practitioner first, especially of you are on blood thinning medications.

Fish or Krill oils will take some time to achieve maximum benefits, so don't expect miracles for at least three months. After that time you should see enough improvement to slowly begin decreasing your prescription medication. Don't do this without medical supervision though!

Green lipped mussel (Lyprinol®)

From the waters of New Zealand, the Green lipped mussel has been hailed as one of the best natural "cures" for rheumatoid arthritis. It has anti-inflammatory properties and some arthritis sufferers swear by it. It does contain a high concentration of Omega 3 fatty acids; however there is no real evidence that the Green lipped mussel is any better than taking fish oil and it is more expensive.

Lyprinol® is the patented marine lipid extract of the shellfish which is composed of a combination of lipid groups and Omega 3 fats. By all means try it, it may well work wonders for you. However do not take if you are allergic to seafood.

Ashwagandha

Ashwagandha is an immune system tonic that also has an overall calming effect. Ashwagandha is used in Ayurvedic medicine and is what's known as an "adaptogen". This means it adapts to the body's needs in a unique way and heals the disorders that it "finds".

This herb is traditionally administered after illness to strengthen the immune system.

Ashwagandha also has anti-inflammatory properties.

Turmeric

Turmeric has numerous health benefits. Turmeric is a bright yellow spice of the ginger family and contains an ingredient called *curcumin*. Although turmeric has strong anti-inflammatory properties, its benefits don't stop there. Curcumin can lower levels of *substance* P (see the section on chronic pain memory) so that fewer pain messages are sent through the nerves.

If you've ever eaten an Indian curry, then you've tasted curcumin. Unfortunately the levels of this ingredient have to be higher to have a therapeutic effect. Aim for 400-600 milligrams a day at least.

As with many of these natural remedies, check with your health care provider if you're taking any type of blood thinning medication.

Cat's claw herb

Cat's claw is a vine that grows in the Amazon rainforest. The bark of the root has been used by the native population for many years for the treatment of ulcers, inflammation and digestive problems. The ingredients in cat's claw can inhibit the body's release of prostaglandins, known to cause inflammation in the body. Cat's claw may also protect cartilage from damage while decreasing the joint pain from rheumatoid arthritis. Cat's claw can also act as an immune system stimulant.

Although further testing is needed, cat's claw is worth a try. You can buy it as a tea or in capsule form and it has few known side effects when taken as prescribed. However don't take if pregnant as it may cause miscarriage. Also check with your doctor if you are taking any prescribed medications.

MSM

MSM is short for *Methylsulfonylmethane*. It is a type of organic sulfur usually associated with the treatment of osteoarthritis. However some people have had remarkable results by taking MSM for rheumatoid arthritis as well. MSM has been claimed to be able to repair damaged body tissues which puts it slightly beyond the role of a temporary pain reliever.

MSM has an anti-inflammatory action and can increase blood supply to the body's tissues. It can also have a relaxing effect on muscles and can ease pain by 80% in some cases. All in all, a useful natural remedy for arthritis of all types.

Vitamins and anti-oxidants

Because today's food supplies can be nutritionally deficient due to over-farming and pesticide use, we tend not to get all our nutritional needs from our diets alone - and that's assuming we eat a healthy diet in the first place! Maintaining good levels of anti-inflammatory vitamins such as Vitamin C and E can really help people with rheumatoid arthritis. Vitamin C is particularly important for maintaining healthy cartilage.

Certain antioxidants can slow cartilage damage and are important if you are taking NSAIDs. Recommended are selenium (don't exceed 200 micrograms), grape seed extract and Lipoic acid. Selenium is toxic in larger doses but is commonly missing in many diets.

Depending on where in the world you're situated, you may be able to get a composite of some of these remedies mixed together in a capsule form. The advantage of trying them separately is to see which ones work for you and which are not effective.

Whatever you decide, make sure the remedies are good quality and all natural with no fillers. Give them a good few weeks before expecting benefits.

I still take Krill oil every day along with a good multi vitamin/mineral supplement. I also take chlorella and enzymes every so often. When I was still experiencing symptoms I took Bromelain and Boswellia. I did try MSM but it didn't agree with me unfortunately.

Points to take away:

- -There are many natural remedies that can ease rheumatoid arthritis pain.

- -Some natural remedies are as effective as chemical pain relieving drugs.

- -Natural remedies by themselves don't have the ability

to reverse the damaged caused by rheumatoid arthritis as far as we know.

WHAT IS THE MOST IMPORTANT ORGAN FOR IMMUNE HEALTH?

The liver is the main detoxification organ of the body. Before toxins can be excreted by the body, they have to be converted into harmless compounds that can be excreted by the kidneys or via the bile.

The liver produces three antioxidants used for this process. *Glutathione*, Co-enzyme *Q10* and *Superoxide dismutase*. These two anti-oxidants and the enzyme work to convert most toxins into a form where they can be released into the bloodstream for elimination.

The liver is extremely efficient, but in can be overwhelmed by chemicals in food and in the environment, such as caffeine, alcohol and medications to name but a few.

What happens when the liver can't keep up with all these chemicals? They get stored in the fat cells of the body, which is like an emergency storage system for anything the body can't process. The necessity of having these fat cells ready to store the toxic overload is one of the reasons we struggle to lose weight, especially around the tummy area. This "belly fat" creates an inflammatory reaction which creates more fat cells and a vicious cycle is created.

As you already know, this is putting a strain on the immune system and predisposing us to immune system disorders, including rheumatoid arthritis. Many studies have been done in recent years to see if there is a link between our modern chemical filled lifestyles and auto-immune diseases. The results up to now have shown a causal link that can't be ignored.

How do we know when our liver is struggling? A blood test will only show damage that has *already* been done, but we want to prevent damage rather than repair it. Here are a few clues that the liver may need some TLC! Don't be too alarmed if you have some of these symptoms, as they can have more than one cause; and anyway we will soon know how to regain a healthy liver.

·A yellowish tinge to the eyes

·Frequent indigestion, especially after eating fatty foods

·Increase in allergies such as hives or hay fever

·Frequent viral infections, such as cold and flu

·Chronic fatigue, or feeling tired all the time

·A rise in LDL cholesterol levels (not necessarily total cholesterol levels)

·A rise in the levels of triglycerides

·A sensitivity to many different foods

·Brown colored blotches on the skin. (These used to be called liver spots)

How can we heal our liver and improve the detoxification process?

We can do this in several ways. Improving our diet will help immensely. Drinking less coffee and alcohol will help too. If you have identified several of the symptoms above, try cutting alcohol out altogether. It won't kill you, honest!

Drink plenty of water, but preferably not out of plastic bottles. Keep a glass of water near you and sip regularly.

Using natural chemical free products to clean your home is another step in the right direction. Avoid using insecticides if possible or see if you can purchase an insecticide made with Pyrethum, which is less toxic.

Use natural beauty products and cosmetics. You can even learn to make your own. Coconut or olive oil, lemons, milk and rose water are good ingredients.

There are also some good supplements which will help keep the liver healthy:

Milk thistle which is also known as St Mary's thistle or *Silymarium*. Milk thistle is a powerful anti-oxidant that also strengthens the outer wall of liver cells to protect them from damage.

Selenium (N.B. This is a micro-nutrient so never exceed the maximum dose).

Co-enzyme Q10 is found in the liver and can also be supplemented. This is particularly important if you are taking any type of medication that lowers cholesterol as this depletes CoQ10.

Dandelion root increases the production of bile in the liver.

Soy lecithin prevents fatty liver and is especially useful for those who drink alcohol.

Alpha lipoic acid helps normalize liver enzymes and boosts Glutathione levels. It protects the liver from free radicals.

Turmeric prevents inflammation of the liver.

Chlorella is green algae, high in chlorophyll, which can be taken in powdered or capsule form. Chlorella has most of the major nutrient groups including protein and is known as one of the "superfoods". Chlorella can neutralize acid in the body (useful for meat eaters) and is also known as an effective detoxing medium. It has been claimed that this algae can remove heavy metals, such as mercury and lead stored in the fat cells.

Start slowly with chlorella as too much too soon can cause digestive upset.

Modified Citrus Pectin (MCP) is another detoxing medium and is frequently used in natural treatments for cancer patients. It also claims to eliminate heavy metals and toxins from the body while leaving beneficial minerals intact. MCP is a powerful immune booster and can also decrease inflammation.

Although the liver needs **Glutathione** to function, taking Glutathione doesn't raise levels. The best way to maintain good Glutathione levels is a good diet and lifestyle. A healthy liver will recycle Glutathione so it can be re-used. Poor lifestyle and dietary habits and aging will slow down this process.

Points to take away:

-The liver is the main detoxification organ in the body.

-An unhealthy liver means an unhealthy immune system.

-A blood test will only reveal significant liver damage.

-We can lessen the chance of liver damage by improving our diet and lifestyle.

-There are supplements that can help support the liver and therefore the immune system.

THE MAGIC OF ENZYMES

Many alternative practitioners are now finding that digestive enzyme supplements can go a lot further than relieving digestive problems. They can also strengthen the immune system, improve circulation and relieve pain, along with many other benefits. More importantly, they can also help relieve the symptoms of rheumatoid arthritis.

You may be wondering why our digestive systems need all this extra help. Well it's partly the diet we eat and partly because, as we age, most of our body systems begin to slow down. The digestive system is no different. Did you know that our bodies are at their peak at the average age of twenty seven? After that there are many bodily systems that begin a gradual decline as we age and one of these is our digestive system. This is due to the slowdown in the production in digestive enzymes by the pancreas which help us digest our food. So what? Well - to simplify - the undigested food particles can leak out of the digestive tract (leaky gut syndrome) and circulate causing inflammation.

There are ways around this of course. One is to eat a high enzyme raw food diet; however this is not really practical in this day and age. The best defense and one I use religiously is *Proteolytic* (protein digesting) enzymes. You can buy these in supplemental form and these enzymes can reduce inflammation, reduce or even halt the symptoms of auto immune disease, help the body heal scar tissue and even prevent heart disease - just to name a few benefits.

Now just to make things more complicated ☺ there are

two kinds of enzymes, digestive and systemic. Digestive enzymes are taken with meals and contain enzymes that help digest food. Systemic are taken between meals and these are the ones I recommend.

Systemic enzymes contain larger amounts of proteolytic enzymes, or protease which have the ability to break down protein. Taken with meals, enzymes can help digest proteins fats and carbohydrates which means the nutritional value in the food is better absorbed.

However taken between meals, protease is no longer needed for digestion and circulates in the bloodstream where it gobbles up undigested proteins and scar tissue (fibrin). Natural practitioners also believe these enzymes can help the breakdown of cancer cells.

Do a search on the web for systemic enzymes. You may want to go into the science a bit more; I have only provided an outline here. However the one I take is called "Neprinol" and it contains all the necessary enzymes needed.

Words of caution, start gradually, or keep a bathroom handy! Slowly increase to the optimal dose.

Points to take away:

- The body makes its own enzymes, but a bad diet and aging means this becomes inefficient.

- Enzyme therapy can stop leaky gut syndrome and improve digestion.

- Proteolytic enzymes consume proteins, such as scar

tissue when not being used for digestion.

ENERGY HEALING FOR RHEUMATOID ARTHRITIS

Energy healing is a rather broad title which includes several modes of healing that vary from the scientific to the esoteric. The main aim of energy healing is to balance all the body's energy to promote optimal health. As it would take several books to outline all the different types of energy therapy, I have outlined the main ones here and also explain the one I used myself.

The Chinese have believed for centuries that we have energy meridians (Chi) running through the body. Western medicine has started to endorse energy therapy by accepting practices such as acupuncture into the main stream of medicine. Homeopathy, Reiki and even prayer can come under this umbrella of holistic remedies.

Energy healing can also heal the condition known as "chronic pain memory". This can be caused by the nerve cells increasing their sensitivity to pain and is something we could all probably do without!

Acupuncture

Acupuncture uses extra thin needles to balance energy and to bring the body to a state of homeostasis. It is a painless procedure and can be tailored to relieve the pain of rheumatoid arthritis. Natural doctors also say that acupuncture triggers the release of endorphins, the body's natural pain killers, which can relieve pain quite effectively. The treatment can last up to an hour and is quite relaxing.

Mainstream medicine is now more accepting of acupuncture and frequently recommends it for the treatment of chronic pain.

Emotional Healing Technique (EFT)

This is the energy healing technique I used and still use today. I started using it when the pain was at its worst and gave up after a few days when it didn't seem to work. I remember feeling rather frustrated as I had been reading all these wonderful cures that people had experienced from EFT, such as healing pain, depression, even long standing illnesses they had experienced for many years. Why didn't it work for me? It wasn't fair!

I then read an article that explained that I had to be persistent with EFT. So I started to try again and promised myself to remember to do it every day. Gradually it formed part of my morning routine and that's when I started noticing results.

So what is EFT? EFT stimulates various meridian points on the body by tapping them with the fingers. This balances the energy in the body and can lead to some surprising results. EFT has been called "acupuncture without needles". It is free, easy to learn, needs no equipment and you don't have to believe in it for it to work ☺

When it was first discovered by a doctor named Roger Callahan, it was assumed that it only healed emotional problems, such as stress, phobias and depression. However it was soon discovered that EFT can work on other diseases which did not appear to have any emotional component.

However most diseases DO have an emotion attached to them, it could be stress or fear or something from childhood. I can't go into this in any great detail here, but I have provided a link to a good EFT article which also has links to a "Get Started" package and other information.

http://bit.ly/ZMhDzk

TENS

TENS is short for *transcutaneous electrical nerve stimulation* which can be used to block pain signals to the brain. It consists of a small machine fitted with sticky pads that pass a very mild electric current onto the skin via small electrodes. This helps block pain signals and can be used on most parts of the body. While not energy healing in the strict sense, I have had a lot of success with TENS and it has saved me from taking pain medication on quite a few occasions.

Nowadays you can get hand-held devices that are battery powered, but still can deliver a strong signal. Place the pads on the painful area and turn the machine on slowly until you can feel a tingling sensation.

TENS, like almost everything, works better for some than for others. I personally did get a lot of relief from it, but others say it is not effective for them. Most physiotherapists use TENS, both for acute and chronic pain.

Points to take away:

-Energy healing encompasses many different healing treatments mainly aimed to bring the energy of the body back into balance.

-Energy healing will work whether you believe in it or not. Treatments such as EFT are free and can be extremely effective. I really suggest you swallow your skepticism and just try it. You may be surprised!

-Energy healing can also eliminate chronic pain memory.

CHRONIC PAIN MEMORY –
WHAT IS IT?

As you are probably well aware, there are two types of pain. Acute pain is sudden - and is the body's warning sign that there is an injury and you have to stop doing whatever it is you're doing! The second type of pain is chronic pain. Chronic pain is persistent and long lasting pain. But there is something you should understand about chronic pain. The pain sensation can change when you have experienced prolonged exposure to it.

Now some people notice a worsening of their pain over time and conclude that their symptoms are getting worse and that the disease is intensifying, however this may not be the case.

This "syndrome" is called *Chronic Pain Memory* or *Neuron Memory*. I hesitate to call it a syndrome because there is an actual physical cause. Chronic pain memory is caused by the chemical pathways behaving abnormally. The nerve cells may increase in sensitivity and the central nervous system fails to control pain sensations as efficiently as it used to.

There is actual scientific proof that this can happen. Magnetic resonance imaging scans of the human brain's *Prefrontal Cortex* area show increased activity in patients who have experienced chronic pain for a long time, compared with those who have no chronic pain. This has not been proven beyond a doubt, but the mounting evidence certainly does point to it.

The cells in the brain also have a "memory". They can recognize a pain that they have felt before and this tends to exaggerate the pain experience. Put all this together with the stress that pain inevitably causes, and we have an unpleasant cycle that develops.

It's now becoming clear that most of us have some memory of pain in our cells whether or not we suffer from painful diseases like arthritis or not. Any pain sensation that lasts for more than a few minutes can leave a memory trace in the cells. These recent findings help us to understand why people who have had limbs amputated, can still "feel" the painful limb.

Then we also have to deal with *Substance P*. Substance P is a neurotransmitter whose function it is to cause pain. Although this is a part of the defense mechanism of the body, we do not need chronic pain messages all day and every day.

Now this may be our body trying to protect us, but, when it comes to a painful disease like rheumatoid arthritis, it's not something we really need! Is there a way around this? Yes!

There are two ways to interrupt this pain pattern; the application of **Capsaicin** to the area can lessen the pain memory trace. You can apply capsaicin cream topically on the painful area or take it in capsule form. A word of warning! This stuff is made from hot chilies and is VERY hot! You may notice a burning sensation for a few days which tends to wear off with time. However do not touch your eyes, nose or mouth until you have washed your hands several times. It's best to wear gloves just in case.

Energy therapy can also erase chronic pain memory when applied properly as it can treat the emotional component of pain. It can do this whether or not you believe in it. Energy therapy is a bit "left field" for some, however trust me, it works! I have used both and energy therapy was the clear winner for me.

We have covered energy therapy in a previous chapter.

There is also a drug called *D-Cycloserine* that has been developed to counter chronic pain memory. This was originally developed for phobias.

Points to take away:

-Pain that lasts for over a few months can cause chronic pain memory, which can intensify the feeling of pain.

-Substance P is a neurotransmitter that causes pain in the body.

-Energy therapy is a valid way to overcome chronic pain memory.

STEM CELL THERAPY

Stem cell therapy is still in its infancy, but there are already exciting discoveries being made. Before we even start on this, I should say that I have no idea how much this would cost in different countries. Probably it would be very expensive! But it's worth considering if you can afford it. Also this may become more affordable as time goes on and it becomes more widespread.

We all have our own stem cells inside our bodies that act as a repair system. As we age, however, the numbers of stem cells in our bodies start to shrink. In the case of auto-immune disease, the stem cells would be overwhelmed with the job of trying to repair damaged joints and tissues, especially in the elderly.

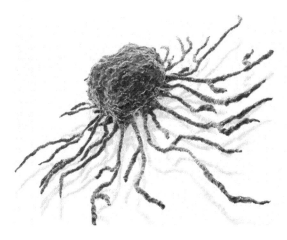

There are two types of stem cells. Human umbilical cord tissue (HUCT) stem cells which are taken from donated umbilical cords and adult stem cells which are taken from your own adipose (fat) tissues. Both these can be very effective. There are also stem cells that are produced from animals, but I really don't know about the suitability of these, especially for those with auto-immune diseases.

The beauty of stem cells is they can develop into different cell types when dividing. A stem cell may become a muscle cell or a skin cell. It could also become a joint cell and this is where it gets exciting for rheumatoid arthritis sufferers!

When stem cells are introduced intravenously to the site of an injury or damaged tissue, they start to repair it by subdividing to replenish damaged cells. At this point in time there is no real way to ensure what type of cell the stem cells will become. They could simply remain as stem cells. The best idea, in the case of rheumatoid arthritis, is to have them injected as near as possible to the affected area.

Another huge advantage of stem cell therapy is that it is unlikely the introduced cells will be rejected by the body. Therefore the need for immune-suppressing drugs is greatly reduced. Adult stem cells are taken from your own body, so they are unlikely to be rejected and HUCT stem cells are not matured so don't seem to trigger an immune response.

Stem cells have been tested for some time on animals and the results have been encouraging. A case in point is the fast repair of injured joints in race horses. The cells are injected into the inflamed joint where they calm inflammation and healing is significantly accelerated. The stem cells also have a benign effect on the immune system while still allowing it to function normally to protect against diseases. They also stimulate the production of T regulatory cells, which can slow the immune attack on the person's own body.

I would suggest finding out more about stem cell therapy if you are interested. There are clinics that do this work, but they may not yet be widely available. Do your homework on them before proceeding. As I've said, this is fairly new and I'm just throwing it in for those who are interested so they can do their own research.

For the average person who can't afford this type of therapy, the best thing to do is to keep your existing stem cells in good condition. The best way to do this is by cutting out smoking, avoiding stress, eating a healthy diet and getting enough sleep. Funny how it always boils down to that, isn't it?

Points to take away:

-Stem cell therapy is effective but may not be
   affordable to everyone.

-You can keep the stem cells in your own body
   healthy.

LOW DOSE NALTREXONE

While Naltrexone is not a natural remedy as such, this particular treatment uses lower doses of this drug and is proving effective against a wide range of auto-immune diseases, including rheumatoid arthritis.

Naltrexone was originally approved for addiction to opium and heroin. Recently, however, it has been found that low doses (1.5 - 4.5 mg) of this medication taken at night, can have beneficial and sometimes immediate effects on symptoms of most auto-immune disorders.

Dr Bernard Bihari was the first to discover alternative uses for low doses of Naltrexone in the US. Although it has been FDA approved for many years for drug addiction, the FDA (at the time of writing) has yet to approve it for the treatment of AIDS, cancer and other auto-immune diseases. People with rheumatoid arthritis who have been treated with LDN have experienced relief from joint pain and swelling.

In simple terms LDN can be effective against auto-immune diseases such as Multiple Sclerosis, Chron's Disease, Alzheimers, Lou Gehrig's Disease, rheumatoid arthritis and many more. It works by restoring the body's natural production of endorphins, thus normalizing the immune system. People with auto-immune disorders generally have a low level of endorphins in their bloodstream.

Naltrexone has been used to treat drug addiction in high

doses (around 50 mg) and is available on a doctor's prescription. However low dose Naltrexone (LDN) is what's needed for immune system treatment and here's the catch. It is not easy to get LDN and it is not necessarily covered by insurance.

However LDN is considered relatively safe, not terribly expensive and there are ways to obtain it. Below is the link to a website (nonprofit) where you can obtain more information on LDN and a list of suppliers. Bear in mind this has not been "officially" tested and approved, but the number of case studies of patients who have had amazing results from this drug for auto-immune conditions continues to rise.

LDN is not a cure and people who stop taking it can have their symptoms return. However it does have very good and fast results without the side effects of some of the other medications prescribed for rheumatoid arthritis pain.

Certainly worth looking into!

For more information, access to LDN and to join a Yahoo! discussion group, visit the link below.

http://www.lowdosenaltrexone.org/

LOOKING AFTER YOURSELF –
A HEALTHY LIFESTYLE

There's not much point in eating a healthy diet and taking the right supplements if your lifestyle is unhealthy. I know, because I did this for many years. I ate a fairly healthy diet and took a multivitamin and exercised regularly. But after each meal I'd go outside and light up a cigarette. Not just after meals either; I smoked around 30 cigarettes a day.

I kidded myself I was doing most things right, so it didn't really matter. I "needed" to smoke to deal with the stress. What I didn't realize was smoking actually causes stress! As nicotine leaves the bloodstream, it causes subtle withdrawal symptoms, until you light up again. Giving up smoking was very hard to do, but one of the best things I have ever done. I thought l couldn't live without cigarettes, but life actually gets better.

Your self-esteem improves as well as your health. Your clothes and breath smell better and your bank balance improves. What's not to like?

Smoking is really bad for your immune system and especially your liver which has to eliminate the many toxins found in cigarette smoke. It's not easy to give it up, but you'll be so glad you did!

Lack of sleep is another immune system depressant. Sometimes we get so busy we just need an extra hour or so a day. Surely cutting out an hour of sleep can't hurt? Believe me it can. Don't let a busy lifestyle interfere with your sleep. You'll achieve so much more when you're well rested!

If you have sleep problems like insomnia, a sleep clinic may be a good idea. They can help to highlight the causes of your sleep problems. Stress is a leading cause of insomnia too. Try yoga or relaxation techniques such as deep breathing to get stress out of your life. It's really bad for your immune system, so do whatever it takes to get rid of stress.

If pain is keeping you awake, then you'll need to tailor your medication so that you're comfortable at night. See your doctor if your pain is worse at night or refer to the chapter on energy therapy. Hopefully when you've implemented some of the suggestions in this book, you'll soon be feeling more comfortable.

Exercise (groan!)

Exercise is crucial for maintaining immune health. Exercise stimulates the lymphatic system to move lymph around the body. It's similar in some ways to the circulatory system, except blood has a pump (the heart) to keep it moving. Lymph is a fluid that travels around the body taking toxins to the elimination points such as the bowels, bladder, skin and lungs. A sluggish lymphatic system can impact on the immune system, so get moving to get rid of those toxins!

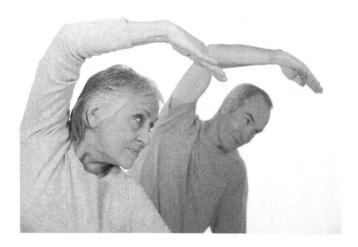

Exercise also strengthens muscles and bones, helps you to lose weight and promotes healthy sleep. Exercise can be difficult when you're experiencing pain, so start gently with walking, swimming or yoga stretches.

Points to take away:

-The following lifestyle habits can affect how your immune system functions:

-Lack of sleep

-Smoking

-Stress

-Lack of exercise

See how many you can address and feel the benefits!

CONCLUSION

I hope you have learned a few things from this book.
Whatever treatment you are on, it's certainly worth striving
to live the healthiest lifestyle that you possibly can. So here
it is again (yes I know you're probably sick of hearing
about it by now...) A healthy diet, plenty of pure water,
plenty of sleep, gentle exercise and avoid stress like the
plague!

I hope that your immune system benefits from the
suggestions and I wish you a long and happy and PAIN
FREE life!

If you have enjoyed this book and feel it has helped you,
could you please return to Amazon and leave a review?
Thank you very much ☺

ABOUT THE AUTHOR

Wendy Owen has a diploma in holistic health and is passionate about natural health, herbal remedies and finding natural answers to cure diseases such as diabetes, insomnia and arthritis among others.

"The body is capable of healing itself given the right environment to do so and I like to help people to be as healthy as they can be, so that disease can be avoided in the first place".

Wendy lives in Queensland Australia, with her husband and small dog.

Made in the USA
Lexington, KY
03 October 2016